Renal Diet Cookbook for Beginners

Regain Control of Your Eating Lifestyle at Every Stage of Kidney Disease with Simple Recipes Low in Sodium, Phosphorus and Potassium

Stephanie Robbins

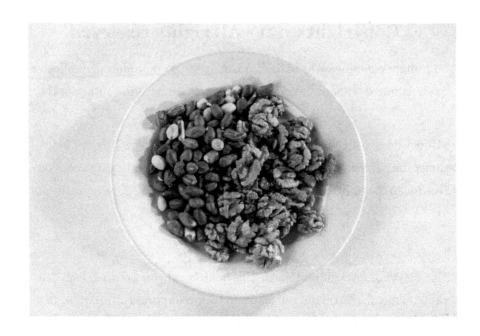

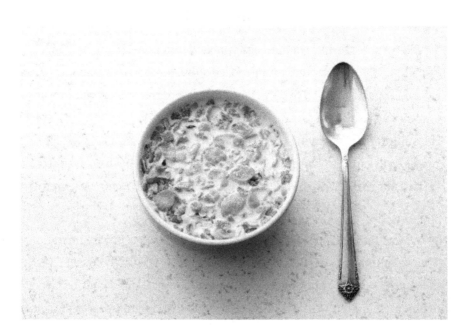

Table of Contents

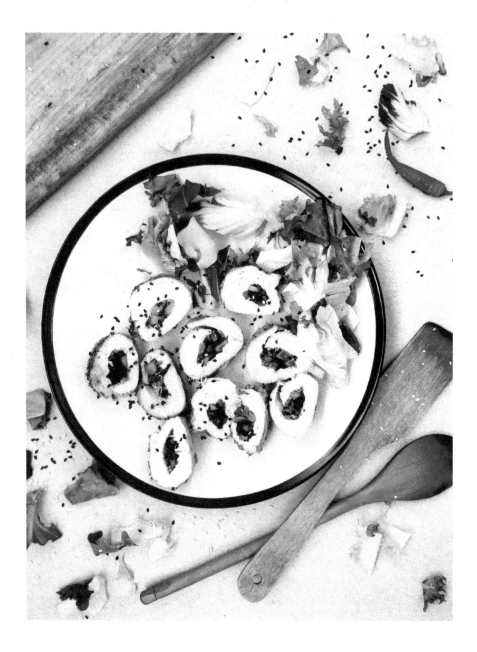

Introduction

To decrease the volume of waste in their blood, individuals with impaired kidney function must stick to a renal or kidney diet. Blood waste occurs from food and drinks that are ingested. As kidney activity is impaired, the kidneys do not filter or extract waste properly. It will adversely influence the electrolyte levels of a patient if excess is left in the blood. Obeying a kidney diet can also help improve kidney function and delay the development of total renal failure.

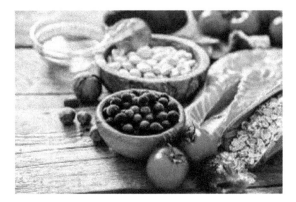

One that is deficient in sodium, phosphorous, and protein is a renal diet.

Renal Diet Essentials

For proper kidney function, eating right is very important. Individuals with kidney illness need to control their potassium, sodium, and phosphorus consumption. Several essential nutrients can need to be regulated by people with kidney illness. The details below will aid you in changing your eating habit. Speak to your doctor or nutritionist regarding your unique and personal food needs.

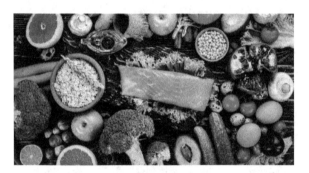

Sodium and Its Role in the Body

Sodium is an inorganic mineral that is contained in most raw foods. The majority of individuals think of salt and sodium as equal. Salt, though, is, in reality, a sodium and chloride complex. The food we consume may include salt, which may contain other sources of sodium. Due to additional salt, refined foods also produce higher sodium levels. Sodium is one of the three main electrolytes of the body (the other two being potassium and chloride). Electrolytes regulate the fluids moving into and out of the tissues and cells of the body. Sodium contributes to:

- Blood pressure and blood flow control

- Nerve activity and muscle contraction regulation

- The control of acid-base blood balance

- Balancing how much fluid is contained or eliminated by the body

Why Should Kidney Patients Control Sodium Consumption?

For patients with renal impairment, too much salt may be dangerous since their kidneys cannot remove extra sodium and fluid from the body properly. As sodium and fluid build-up in the bloodstream and tissues, they can cause:

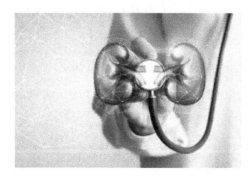

- Heightened thirst

- Swelling in the thighs, hands, and face: edema

- Blood Pressure fluctuation

- Heart failure: The heart will overwork with extra fluid in the bloodstream, rendering it enlarged and sluggish.

- Shortness of breath: Fluid in the lungs will build up, making it hard to breathe.

Ways to Reduce Sodium Intake

- When preparing meals, do not add salt.

- When you eat, don't add extra salt to the food.

- Make a habit of reading the labeling on foods. Stop foods having more than 300 mg of sodium per meal (or 600 mg for a wholly frozen meal). For the first 5 to 6 products of the product list, stop things that contain salt.

- Do not consume bacon, ham, hot dogs, sausages, meat, or nuggets for lunch, or daily condensed soup. Feed only soups that must have logos that decrease your sodium level-and use only a cup-not the entire can.

- Preserved vegetables need to claim "no extra salt."

- Do not include salts like onion salt, garlic salt, or 'seasoned' salt flavored. Stop kosher or some sea salt as well.

- Do not buy "placed in some kind of solution" processed refrigerated or frozen meats, or pre-seasoned / spiced. Chicken breasts, pork chops, pork tenderloin, steaks, or burgers are typically those products.

Potassium and Its Role in the Body

Potassium is an inorganic mineral present in all of the things that we consume and is found primarily in the body as well. Potassium plays a large part in holding the pulse regularly and the muscles functioning properly. For the preservation of fluid and electrolyte equilibrium in the bloodstream, potassium is also required. The kidneys help you keep the body's proper potassium level and remove excessive levels into the urine.

Why Should Kidney Patients Control Potassium Consumption?

They will no longer expel surplus potassium as the kidneys malfunction, so potassium levels build up in your body. High blood potassium is recognized as hyperkalemia, which may prompt:

- Heart attacks

- Slow pulse

- An irregular heartbeat

- Muscle weakness

- Death

Ways to Reduce Potassium Intake

- Speak regarding developing a meal schedule with a renal dietitian.

- Limit items with a strong potassium content.

- Limit food items and milk to 8 oz a day.

- Choose fruits and vegetables that are fresh.

- Stop sodium substitutes & potassium seasonings.

- Learn to label & stop potassium chloride on processed goods.

- To serve scale, pay attention.

- Hold your diet diary.

Potassium-rich diets to sidestep

- Winter squash

- Pumpkin

- Dried beans – all kinds

- Tomatoes, tomato sauce, tomato juice

- Prune juice

- Grapefruit juice

- Oranges and orange juice

- Bananas

Phosphorous and Its Role in the Body

Phosphorus is a mineral essential in the preservation and growth of bones. Phosphorus frequently helps grow connective tissue and organs and assists in the movement of muscles. As phosphorus-containing food is eaten and digested, phosphorus is removed by the small intestines such that it can be contained in the bones.

Why Should Kidney Patients Control Phosphorous Consumption?

Normal functioning kidneys can extract excess phosphorus from the blood. The kidneys no longer expel surplus phosphorus while kidney activity is impaired. High levels of phosphorus can pull calcium from one's bones, making them fragile. This often results in toxic calcium concentrations in the blood vessels, lungs, skin, and heart.

Ways to Control Phosphorus Intake

- The diet's primary phosphorus source is dairy goods, so restrict milk to a cup each day. Just one glass OR 1 ounce a day, whether you use cheese or yogurt in the place of condensed milk!

- Phosphorus is also present in certain vegetables. Avoid the greens, dried beans, mushrooms, broccoli, and Brussels sprouts to 1 cup each WEEK.

- Also, the patient needs to restrict the mentioned cereals to one serving per week: wheat cereals, bran, oatmeal, and granola.

- White bread is safer than bread or crackers of whole grains.

- There is phosphorus in soft drinks but consume just one time. Do not consume Dr. Pepper ® (any type), colas, Mountain Dew ® (any type), and root beers. Hawaiian Punch ®, Fruit works ®, Cool ® iced tea, and Aquafina ® tangerine pineapple are also prevented.

Chapter 1: Breakfast Recipes

1. Sausage and Egg Sandwich

Serves: 1

Prep time: 5 min

Cooking time: 5 min

Ingredients:

- 1 tbsp shredded cheddar cheese

- 1 patty of turkey sausage

- ¼ cup liquid egg substitute – low cholesterol

- 1 English muffin

- Cooking spray

Directions:

1. Spray a tiny saucepan with oil and heat it.

2. Pour in and heat the egg replacer, turning it nearly through as heated.

3. Toast the muffin with toast.

4. Patty is baked in the oven.

5. Fold the egg and put it, covered with the patty, in the muffin.

6. Sprinkle with cheese, top up with the top of the muffin and eat.

2. Homemade Granola

Serves: 10

Prep time: 10 min

Cooking time: 30-40 min

Ingredients:

- 300g (10½oz) rolled oats

- 2 tbsp of soft brown sugar

- 1 tbsp of lemon juice

- 2 tbsp of clear honey or golden syrup

- 4 tbsp of sunflower or vegetable oil

- Dried cranberries (optional)

Directions:

1. Preheat your oven to about 140°C/275°F.

2. The oil, honey/syrup, lemon juice and sugar are melted in a wide saucepan over medium heat. The goal is not to cause the mix to boil, only to allow the ingredients to melt and blend together. Then add the oats and whisk thoroughly.

3. Spread the mixture in an even layer on a baking tray (depending on their height, you will need two baking trays. Bake in the oven until crisp for around 30-40 min. Check the granola every 10 min and swirl to ensure an even bake.

4. You could add a few handfuls of dried cranberries until cooked and chilled. The granola can be placed in an airtight jar and used within one month.

3. Festive Berry Parfait

Serves: 4

Prep time: 20 min plus 1 hour for chilling

Cooking time: None

Ingredients:

- 1 cup sliced fresh strawberries

- 2 cup fresh blueberries

- 1 cup crumbled Meringue Cookies

- ½ tsp ground cinnamon

- 1 tbsp granulated sugar

- ½ cup plain cream cheese, at room temperature

- 1 cup vanilla rice milk, at room temperature

Directions:

1. Whisk the milk, sugar, cream cheese, and cinnamon together in a small cup until creamy.

2. Spoon ¼ cup of the crumbled cookie into 4 (6-ounce) glasses at the bottom of each.

3. On top of the cakes, spoon ¼ cup of the cream cheese mixture.

4. Place ¼ cup of the berries on top of the cream cheese.

5. Repeat with the cookies, cream cheese mix, and berries in each cup.

6. For 1 hour, cool in the fridge and serve.

4. Baked Egg Cup

Serves: 12

Prep time: 10 min

Cooking time: 25 min

Ingredients:

- 12 eggs

- ¼ tsp black pepper

- 1/3 cup mushrooms

- 1/3 cup bell pepper

- 1/3 cup of onion

- 6 slices of bacon, low sodium

Directions:

1. Preheat your oven to about 350°F and use paper liners to fill a muffin tray.

2. Dice all of the veggies and cook your bacon and crumble them into the veggies.

3. Put your blend into the cup.

4. Beat and add the eggs and pepper into the cup, allowing a little room in each one.

5. Bake the muffins for around 25 min or before they grow and firm up.

6. Serve it warm.

5. Healthy Porridge

Serves: 4

Prep time: 4-5 min

Cooking time: 1-2 min

Ingredients:

- Sprinkle of cinnamon

- ½ grated apple

- 100ml water

- 100ml skimmed milk

- 35g (1¼oz) porridge oats

Directions:

1. In a pot, combine all the ingredients, warm the pan and boil for about 3-4 min.

2. Alternatively, cook for about 1-2 min in the microwave, stirring at intervals of 30 seconds.

6. Watermelon-Raspberry Smoothie

Serves: 2

Prep time: 10 min

Cooking time: None

Ingredients:

- 1 cup ice

- ½ cup fresh raspberries

- 1 cup diced watermelon

- ½ cup boiled, cooled, and shredded red cabbage

Directions:

1. In a mixer, put the cabbage and pump for 2 min or until it is finely chopped.

2. Add in the watermelon and raspberries and pulse until quite well mixed, or around 1 min.

3. Until the smoothie is very rich and smooth, add the ice and mix.

4. Pour into 2 glasses and serve.

7. Apple Fritter Rings

Serves: 20

Prep time: 5 min

Cooking time: 1-2 min

Ingredients:

- ½ tsp cinnamon

- ¾ cup oil for deep frying

- 1 tsp canola oil

- 1/3 cup almond milk

- 1/3 cup low-fat 1% milk

- 1 beaten egg

- 1 tsp baking powder

- 6 tbsp sugar

- 1 cup white flour

- 4 large cooking apples

Directions:

1. Peel and core the apples. From each apple, cut 5 circles, 1⁄2 "thick.

2. Sift together the rice, baking powder and two tsp of sugar together.

3. In a separate dish, combine the egg, almond yogurt, milk, and 1 tsp of oil.

4. Combine the egg and dried mixtures before they are combined.

5. In a deep skillet, boil an inch of cooking oil.

6. Dip the apple rings in the batter and fried until golden brown or for 1 to 1 1⁄2 min.

7. Drain them on towels made of cloth.

8. Combine the remaining sugar with the cinnamon and scatter over the patties.

8. High Energy Porridge

Serves: 4

Prep time: 15-20 min

Cooking time: 15 min

Ingredients:

- 200ml full-fat milk

- 35g (1¼oz) porridge oats

- Optional: add some cream and syrup or jam for additional energy

Directions:

1. In a pan, combine all the ingredients, heat the pan and boil the mix for about 3-4 min.

2. Or you may cook for about 1-2 min in a microwave, stirring at intervals of 30 seconds.

9. Blueberry-Pineapple Smoothie

Serves: 2

Prep time: 15 min

Cooking time: None

Ingredients:

- ½ cup of water

- ½ apple

- ½ cup English cucumber

- ½ cup pineapple chunks

- 1 cup frozen blueberries

Directions:

1. In a mixer, add the blueberries, cucumber, pineapple, apple, and water and combine until thick and creamy.

2. Pour the smoothie into 2 glasses and enjoy.

10. The Beach Boy Omelete

Serves: 1

Prep time: 5 min

Cooking time: 5-10 min

Ingredients:

- 2 sprigs parsley

- 1 tbsp soy milk

- 2 egg whites

- 1 whole egg

- 2 tbsp shredded frozen hash browns

- 2 tbsp diced green bell pepper

- 2 tbsp diced onion

- 1 tsp canola oil

Directions:

1. Heat the oil and add the onion and pepper. Sauté for approximately 2 min.

2. Add in the browns with shredded hash and simmer for another 5 min.

3. Whip the milk and eggs and dump the mixture into a separate Omelet tray.

4. Cook until your Omelet is solid.

5. Place the hash brown mixture in the Omelet center and roll up the Omelet.

6. Garnished with new parsley for serving.

11. Traditional Cooked English breakfast

Serves: 1

Prep time: 5 min

Cooking time: 5 min

Ingredients:

- 4 small mushrooms or 1 small tomato, or 2 tbsp of baked beans

- 2 pieces of bacon or 1 sausage (remove fat or opt for low fat if trying to lose weight)

- As much toast as you like (although be careful if you are trying to lose weight)

- 1 egg – any way you like

Directions:

If you are attempting to lose weight, so grilling is the safest way of cooking, or you may fry with minimum oil in a non-stick frying pan or use spray oil. Then frying in fat can help raise the calories in your breakfast if you need to add weight.

12. Apple-Chai Smoothie

Serves: 2

Prep time: 5 min, plus 30 min to steep

Cooking time: 5 min

Ingredients:

- 2 cup ice

- 1 apple, peeled, cored, and chopped

- 1 chai tea bag

- 1 cup unsweetened rice milk

Directions:

1. Warm the rice milk in a large saucepan over low-medium heat for around 5 min or until steaming.

2. Remove the milk from the flame and steeply add the teabag.

3. Let the milk cool for approximately 30 min in the fridge with the teabag, and then remove the teabag, squeezing gently to release all the taste.

4. In a blender, put the milk, apple, and ice and blend until smooth.

5. Pour it into 2 glasses and serve.

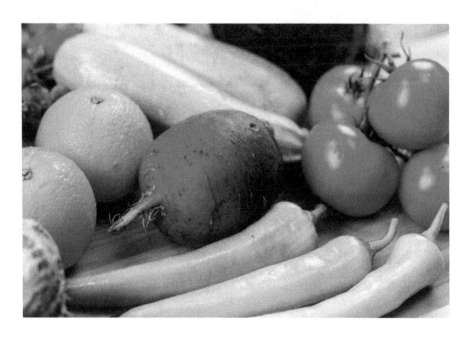

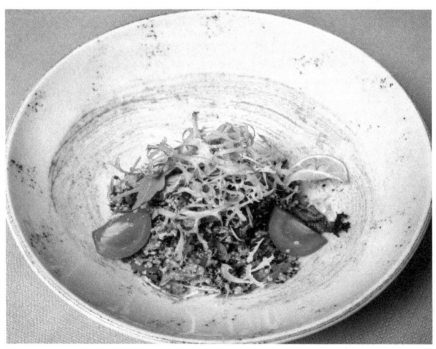

Chapter 2: Lunch/Dinner Recipes

13. Strawberry Watercress Salad with Almond Dressing

Serves: 6

Prep time: 15 min

Cooking time: None

Ingredients:

For the dressing

- Freshly ground black pepper

- ¼ tsp ground mustard

- ¼ tsp pure almond extract

- 1 tbsp honey

- ¼ cup of rice vinegar

- ¼ cup olive oil

For the salad

- 1 cup sliced strawberries

- ½ English cucumber, chopped

- ½ red onion, sliced very thin

- 2 cup shredded green leaf lettuce

- 2 cup roughly chopped watercress

Directions:

Dressing

1. Mix the olive oil and rice vinegar together in a tiny bowl until it is emulsified.

2. Add in some honey, almond extract, mustard, and pepper to the whisk; set aside.

Salad

1. Simply throw the cress, green leaf lettuce, onion, cucumber, and strawberries together in a large cup.

2. Over the salad, pour the dressing and mix to blend.

14. Leaf Lettuce and Carrot Salad with Balsamic Vinaigrette

Serves: 4

Prep time: 25 min

Cooking time: None

Ingredients:

For the vinaigrette

- Freshly ground black pepper

- Pinch red pepper flakes

- 2 tbsp chopped fresh oregano

- 4 tbsp balsamic vinegar

- ½ cup olive oil

For the salad

- 3 large radishes, sliced thin

- ¾ cup fresh green beans, cut into 1-inch pieces

- 1 carrot, shredded

- 4 cup shredded green leaf lettuce

Directions:

Vinaigrette

1. Mix together the balsamic vinegar, olive oil, oregano, and red pepper flakes in a tiny cup.

2. Add spice seasoning.

Salad

1. Add the carrot, lettuce, green beans, and radishes together in a wide cup.

2. Add the vegetables to the vinaigrette and toss to cover them.

3. To eat, set the salad on four plates.

15. Grilled Salmon with a Herb Crust

Serves: 4

Prep time: 15 min

Cooking time: 30 min

Ingredients:

- ¼ tsp black pepper

- 1 tbsp olive oil

- 1 tbsp lemon juice

- 1 clove of garlic

- 1/3 cup cilantro

- ¼ cup green onion

- ½ cup oregano

- 4 salmon fillets, skinless

- ¼ tsp salt

Directions:

1. Preheat the oven to a temperature of 400°F.

2. Use aluminum foil to create a pocket for any fillet.

3. Chop up the cilantro, oregano, onion, and garlic and combine in a blender or food processor with the lemon juice, salt, pepper, and olive oil.

4. Coat the mixture with salmon and lock it in the bag.

5. Bake for 30 min or until the salmon is completely cooked.

16. Honey Glazed Pork or Lamb Chops

Serves: 2

Prep time: 15 min

Cooking time: 15 min

Ingredients:

- Black pepper

- 1 tsp wholegrain mustard

- 1 tsp honey

- 25g (¾oz) butter or low-fat spread

- 2 lamb or pork chops

Directions:

1. Beat or scatter the butter until smooth.

2. Mix the mustard and honey and season with the pepper and mix to make a smooth paste. For approximately an hour, brush the honey mixture over your picked chop, cover and relax. Grill the chops on each side under a hot grill for 5 min until cooked and eat.

17. Minted Lamb Chops

Serves: 2

Prep time: 15 min

Cooking time: 15 min

Ingredients:

- 1 tbsp of vegetable or olive oil

- 1 free-range egg, whisked

- 100g (3½oz) flour

- 2 lamb chops

- 1 tbsp fresh parsley

- 2 tbsp fresh mint

- 100g (3½oz) breadcrumbs (homemade or shop brought)

Directions:

1. Use a mixer to incorporate the breadcrumbs, mint and parsley until well mixed to cook the lamb chops. Set it in a container.

2. Cover the lamb chops in the starch, and then dip until well covered in the egg and into the breadcrumbs, and add spice seasoning.

3. Heat a medium-hot frying pan. Place the lamb chops in the pan and add the grease. For three min, cook.

4. Switch over the chops and simmer for three more min.

5. Remove the chops and allow them to relax, and then serve for three min.

18. Chicken and Lemon Casserole

Serves: 4

Prep time: 15-20 min

Cooking time: 1hour

Ingredients:

- 500ml hot low salt chicken stock

- 2 tbsp honey

- 4 garlic cloves crushed

- 1 tbsp of vegetable or olive oil

- 80g (3oz) butter

- salt and freshly ground black pepper

- 2kg (4lb/4oz) skinless chicken thighs or drumsticks

- 1 lemon, zest and juice only, plus one lemon, sliced into thin rounds

- 2 tsp of dried thyme (optional)

Directions:

1. Preheat the oven to about 200°C/400°F.

2. In a cup, put the sugar, lemon zest and lemon juice and whisk until well blended. Add the bits of chicken and switch until they are thoroughly covered in the mixture. Put aside to marinate for at least 10 min.

3. Heat 40g/1½ oz of butter and half of the olive oil in a flame-proof casserole pan over medium heat. Add half the marinated chicken parts and fried for 5-6 min while the butter is foaming, regularly rotating, until golden-brown. With the remaining butter oil and chicken parts, set the chicken pieces aside, repeat the operation, and then set the chicken aside.

4. Add to the pan the garlic cloves, lemon slices and leftover marinade juices and mix well, wiping a wooden spoon off any burnt pieces from the bottom of the pan. Return the pieces of cooked chicken to the tub, then add the thyme and the hot chicken stock and mix well. Carry

the mixture to a boil and roast in the oven for 30-35 min, or until the chicken is cooked and tender.

5. Remove the pieces of chicken from the pan and put them aside on a warm plate. Strain the sauce through a fine sieve into a saucepan, using the back of a wooden spoon to press the garlic pulp through the sieve. Simmer the lemon sauce for another 5-10 min over high heat or until the liquid is reduced to a thin syrup consistency.

6. Spoon over the casseroled chicken with lemon sauce and eat.

19. Farfalle Confetti Salad

Serves: 6

Prep time: 30 min plus 1 hour for chilling

Cooking time: None

Ingredients:

- Freshly ground black pepper.

- ½ tsp granulated sugar

- 1 tsp chopped fresh parsley

- 1 tbsp freshly squeezed lemon juice

- ½ cup Homemade Mayonnaise

- ½ scallion, green part only, finely chopped

- 2 tbsp yellow bell pepper

- ¼ cup grated carrot

- ¼ cup finely chopped cucumber

- ¼ cup boiled and finely chopped red bell pepper

- 2 cup cooked farfalle pasta

Directions:

1. Toss the pasta, cucumber, red pepper, yellow pepper, carrot, and scallion together in a wide pot.

2. Whisk together the lemon juice, mayonnaise, parsley, and sugar in a shallow pot.

3. For the pasta mixture, add the dressing and whisk to blend. And spice seasoning.

4. Until serving, cool your salad in the refrigerator for at least 1 hour.

20. Couscous Salad with Spicy Citrus Dressing

Serves: 6

Prep time: 25 min plus 1 hour for chilling

Cooking time: None

Ingredients:

For the dressing

- Freshly ground black pepper.

- Pinch cayenne pepper

- Zest of 1 lime

- Juice of 1 lime

- 1 tbsp chopped fresh parsley

- 3 tbsp freshly squeezed grapefruit juice

- ¼ cup olive oil

For the salad

- 1 apple, cored and chopped

- 1 scallion, both white and green parts, chopped

- ½ red bell pepper, chopped

- 3 cup cooked couscous, chilled

Directions:

To make the dressing

1. Mix the grapefruit juice, olive oil, lime zest, lime juice, parsley, and cayenne pepper together in a shallow dish.

2. Add black pepper to season.

To make the salad

1. Blend together the red pepper, chilled couscous, scallion and apple in a wide dish.

2. For the couscous mixture, add the dressing and toss to blend.

3. Until serving, cool your salad in the fridge for at least 1 hour.

21. Shepherd's Pie

Serves: 4

Prep time: 10 min

Cooking time: 40-45 min

Ingredients:

- ½ cup beef gravy

- 1 cup milk, 1%

- 2 tsp Worcestershire sauce

- ½ tsp black pepper

- 2 potatoes

- 1 ½ lb. ground beef

- 4 tbsp butter

- 1/3 cup tomato sauce

- 3 garlic cloves

- ¾ cup frozen peas

- 1 onion

- ¾ cup carrot

Directions:

1. Dice the onion and carrot and mince the garlic as well.

2. Peel and carve the potatoes into cubes of ½.

3. For around 5 min, boil the potatoes, rinse and repeat until the potatoes are soft.

4. In a skillet, melt half of the butter and fry the garlic and onion for around 10 min.

5. Stir in the beef and sauté until it's orange.

6. Add the sauce, pepper, onions and tomato sauce from Worcestershire.

7. For about 10 min, cook uncovered

8. Preheat the oven to 400°F.With the remainder of the butter, scramble the potatoes and blend the milk in. Season using black pepper.Spread the beef and top with the potato in a baking tray. Bake for about 30 min, until bubbly. Serve with some gravy.

22. Apple Pork Chops with Stuffing

Serves: 6 portions

Prep time: 10 min

Cooking time: 45 min

Ingredients:

- 6 pork loin chops, boneless

- 20 oz apple pie filling

- 2 tbsp margarine, unsalted

- 6 oz low-sodium stuffing mix

Directions:

1. Preheat your oven to about 350°F.

2. Spray oil on a pan of 9x13 inches.

3. Through applying water and margarine to the blend and mixing thoroughly, render the stuffing; set aside.

4. Pour the pie filling over the pan's base and place the pork chops on top of the pan.

5. Cover with aluminum foil and bake for approximately 30 min.

6. Remove the foil; cook for the next 10 min and serve once warmed.

23. Chicken or Vegetarian Curry

Serves: 4

Prep time: 5-10 min

Cooking time: 15-20 min

Ingredients:

- 150ml cream

- 1 tsp soft dark brown sugar

- 2 tbsp mango chutney

- 300ml of chicken or vegetable stock

- ½ tsp powdered ginger

- 1 medium onion

- 2 tbsp cooking oil

- 450g chicken in 2.5 cm cubes or 400g tin of chickpeas

Seasoning

- 1 tsp ground cumin

- 1 tsp ground coriander

- 1 tbsp hot curry powder (use mild if you prefer)

- 1 tbsp turmeric

- 1 tsp chili powder

- 1 tsp cayenne pepper (less if you are not keen on a hot curry or omit completely)

- 1 tsp paprika

- 55g plain flour (useless is making with Chickpeas e.g., 25g)

Directions:

1. Mix in a bowl the spice ingredients together and then add to cover the chicken or chickpeas.

2. In a big heavy saucepan, heat the oil, add the chicken or chickpeas and cook until it is sealed.

3. Add in the ginger and onion and simmer for another 1-2 min.

4. Connect the stock, sugar, chutney, and bring it to a simmer. Cover and cook for 15 min, then set aside.

5. Stir in the milk and cook up, taking note that the sauce does not simmer.

6. Serve with boiled rice and some veggies, preferably brown rice.

24. Chicken and Olive Casserole

Serves: 4

Prep time: 150 min

Cooking time: 1 hour

Ingredients:

- Pepper

- 2 tsp balsamic vinegar

- 800g (1lb 8oz) chicken breast

- ½ tsp sugar

- 2 cloves garlic, minced

- 1 tsp dried sage

- 375ml low salt chicken stock

- ½ tsp dried thyme

- 400g tin of chopped tomatoes

- 1 large onion, sliced

- 1 cup olives in brine (black or green or a mixture)

Chapter 3: Starters, Soups and Snacks

25. Roasted Onion Garlic Dip

Serves: 6

Prep time: 15 min plus 1-hour chill time

Cooking time: 1 hour

Ingredients:

- Freshly ground black pepper

- 1 tsp chopped fresh thyme

- 1 tbsp chopped fresh parsley

- 1 tbsp fresh lemon juice

- ½ cup light sour cream

- 2 tsp olive oil

- 8 garlic cloves

- 1 large sweet onion, peeled and cut into eighths

Directions:

1. Preheat your oven to about 425°F.

2. Add your onion and garlic with the olive oil in a shallow pot.

3. To a piece of aluminum foil, move the onion and garlic and loosely bundle the vegetables in a packet.

4. Place a small baking sheet with the foil packet and place the sheet in the oven.

5. Roast the vegetables, or until they are very fragrant and yellow, for 50 min to 1 hour.

6. Take the packet out of the oven and let it cool for 15 min.

7. Stir the lemon juice, sour cream, thyme, parsley, and black pepper together in a medium dish.

8. Carefully open the foil package and pass the vegetables onto a cutting board.

9. Cut the vegetables and add them to the mix with sour cream. Stir to blend.

10. Until serving, wrap the dip and chill in the fridge for about an hour.

26. Chicken Noodle Soup

Serves: 1

Prep time: 15 min

Cooking time: 25 min

Ingredients:

- 2 oz uncooked egg noodles

- ¼ cup carrot

- 1 cup cooked chicken

- ¼ tsp poultry seasoning

- ¼ tsp black pepper

- ¼ tsp salt

- 1 cup of water

- 1 ½ cup chicken broth, low-sodium

Directions:

1. In a slow cooker, place the water and broth and transform the heat to high.

2. Adding salt, pepper, and seasoning for poultry.

3. Dice the carrot and shred the chicken into bits.

4. Add the noodles to your soup.

5. Cook on high flame for around 25 min or until the pasta is ready.

27. Goat's Cheese Rarebit

Serves: 2

Prep time: 15 min

Cooking time: 25 min

Ingredients:

- 4 slices bread

- 2 egg yolks

- ½ tsp mustard

- 25g (¾oz) flour

- 175g (6oz) soft goat's cheese

- pepper

- 150ml soya milk (we used unsweetened)

- 25g (¾oz) olive oil, vegetable spread or butter

Directions:

1. In a saucepan, put the soya milk, spread or butter, cheese, and heat gently until melted and creamy.

2. Mix the flour in and put the mixture to a boil, stirring continuously as it thickens.

3. Remove from the flame and add in the mustard and pepper. Let it rest for 5 min to cool, then stir in the egg yolks with a fork.

4. On the one hand, toast the bread, turn around, and cut the slices' rarebit blend.

5. Put under a hot grill and grill until golden and fizzing.

28. Baba Ganoush

Serves: 6

Prep time: 20 min

Cooking time: 30 min

Ingredients:

- 1 tbsp lemon juice

- 1 tsp ground coriander

- 1 tsp ground cumin

- 2 garlic cloves, halved

- 1 large sweet onion, peeled and diced

- 1 tbsp olive oil, plus extra for brushing

- Freshly ground black pepper

- 1 medium eggplant, halved and scored with a crosshatch pattern on the cut sides

Directions:

1. Preheat your oven to about 400°F.

2. Line 2 baking sheets with some parchment paper.

3. Rub the eggplant halves with some olive oil and put them on one baking sheet, cut-side-down.

4. Mix the garlic, one tbsp of olive oil, onion, cumin, and cilantro together in a shallow dish.

5. On the other baking sheet, scatter the seasoned onions.

6. Put both baking sheets in the oven, roast the onions for 20 min or until softened and browned, and the eggplant for 30 min.

7. Scrape the eggplant flesh into a bowl and cut the vegetables from the oven.

8. To a cutting board, move the onions and garlic and chop coarsely; Add to the eggplant.

9. Stir in the spice and lemon juice.

10. Serve chilled or hot.

29. Grilled PBJ Sandwich

Serves: 2

Prep time: 15 min

Cooking time: 25 min

Ingredients:

- 2 tsp unsalted butter

- 2 tbsp peanut butter

- 1 tbsp jelly

- 2 slices of fresh white bread

Directions:

1. Heat up your frying pan.

2. Butter your bread.

3. Spread some peanut butter and the jelly on the unbuttered sides of the bread.

4. Take your sandwich and put it in the hot skillet.

5. Grill each side until slightly dark.

30. Pesto Cream Veggie Dip

Serves: 2

Prep time: 15 min

Cooking time: 25 min

Ingredients:

- 2 tbsp parmesan cheese

- 100g (3½oz) sour cream

- 100g (3½oz) cream cheese

- 200g (7oz) basil pesto

Directions:

1. Place the cream cheese, pesto, sour cream, and Parmesan cheese and mix well in a cup.

2. Mix until creamy and chill until ready to serve.

31. Cheese-Herb Dip

Serves: 8

Prep time: 15-20 min

Cooking time: None

Ingredients:

- ¼ tsp freshly ground black pepper

- ½ tsp chopped fresh thyme

- 1 tsp minced garlic

- 1 tbsp freshly squeezed lemon juice

- 1 tbsp chopped fresh basil

- 1 tbsp chopped fresh parsley

- ½ scallion, green part only, finely chopped

- ½ cup unsweetened rice milk

- 1 cup cream cheese

Directions:

1. Add the milk, cream cheese, parsley, scallion, lemon juice, basil, thyme, garlic, and pepper together in a medium bowl until well blended.

2. Place the dip for up to 1 week in a sealed jar in the fridge.

32. Egg Sausage Soup

Serves: 1 ½ cup

Prep time: 15 min

Cooking time: 20 min

Ingredients:

- 4 tbsp fresh parsley

- 1 ½ cup water

- 3 cup chicken broth, low-sodium

- 2 whole garlic cloves

- 1 tbsp low-sodium seasoning blend

- 2 tbsp extra virgin olive oil

- 4 slices of bread

- ½ tsp garlic powder

- ½ tsp dried basil

- ½ tsp ground sage

- ½ tsp black pepper

- 4 eggs

- ½ lb. ground beef

- 2 tbsp parmesan cheese, grated

Directions:

1. Preheat your oven to about 375°F.

2. In a pot, combine the meat, garlic powder, basil, pepper, and sage and set it on one side.

3. Dice the bread into 1-inch cubes and toss in the olive oil and seasoning combination. Bake for about 8 min, until lightly browned.

4. In a skillet, crumble the sausage and fry until fried. Drain it on some paper towels.

5. Keep up to 2 tbsp in a separate bowl. Mince the garlic and sauté for around 1 to 2 min after dripping from the plate.

6. Top the skillet with the minced parsley, broth and water and carry to a simmer.

7. Reduce the flame and simmer for around 10 min, then crank up the heat such that the broth just cooks.

8. Crack the eggs into a cup one at a time and slide them into the broth.

9. For around 3 min or until the eggs are placed, poach.

10. Divide the sausage into four bowls, pass the eggs to the bowls using a slotted spoon, and then spill one broth cup into the bowls.

11. With the croutons and parmesan egg, finish off.

33. Smoked Mackerel Pate

Serves: 1-6

Prep time: 15 min

Cooking time: 25 min

Ingredients:

- 1 tbsp creamed horseradish

- 100g (3½oz) cream cheese

- 1 lemon

- 2 spring onions, trimmed and finely sliced

- 200g (7oz) smoked mackerel fillets, skin removed

- Pepper

Directions:

1. Split the mackerel into pieces and cut it finely.

2. Add the cream cheese, mackerel, creamed horseradish, spring onions, and one lemon zest to a bowl and blend.

3. Squeeze the zester lemon juice into it, and blend again until the paste is coarse.

4. Season with pepper to taste.

34. Baking Powder Biscuits

Serves: 2

Prep time: 15 min

Cooking time: 25 min

Ingredients:

- ½ cup of water
- ¼ cup 1% milk
- ⅓ cup vegetable shortening
- 2 tsp sugar
- 3 tsp double-acting baking powder
- 2 cup all-purpose flour, sifted

Directions:

1. Pre-heat the oven to 350°F.

2. Sift into a tub of dry ingredients.

3. Shorten and cut before coarse crumbs develop. In the mixture, make a well.

4. Through the well, add milk and water.

5. With a fork, stir rapidly before the dough leads the fork across the cup.

6. It should be fluffy in the dough. On a well-floured board, spin the dough.

7. 10-12 times, knead softly. Until ½ inch thick, curl or pat dough.

8. In the starch, dip a 2 ½ inch biscuit cutter, then cut out 10 biscuits.

9. For 12-15 min, bake the biscuits on an ungreased baking dish.

35. Spicy Kale Chips

Serves: 6

Prep time: 15-20 min

Cooking time: 25 min

Ingredients:

- Pinch cayenne pepper

- ¼ tsp chili powder

- 2 tsp olive oil

- 2 cup kale

Directions:

1. Preheat the oven to 300°F.

2. Line 2 parchment paper baking sheets; set aside.

3. From the kale, cut the stems and break the leaves into 2-inch parts.

4. Wash the kale and thoroughly dry it.

5. To a wide cup, switch the kale and drizzle with olive oil.

6. To toss the kale with the oil, use your palms, making sure to coat each leaf uniformly.

7. To mix thoroughly, season the kale with chili powder and cayenne pepper and toss.

8. Spread the seasoned kale on each baking sheet in a single layer. The leaves should not match.

9. Cook the kale, turning the pans once, for 20 to 25 min or until the kale is dry and crisp.

10. Remove the trays from the oven and give 5 min for the chips to chill on the trays.

11. Instantly serve.

36. Yucatan Lime Soup

Serves: 1 ½ cup

Prep time: 10 min

Cooking time: 10-15 min

Ingredients:

- 1/1 tsp black pepper

- ¼ cup fresh squeezed lime juice

- ¼ cup fresh chopped cilantro

- 1 whole bay leaf

- ¼ tsp salt

- 4 cup chicken broth, low-sodium,

- Cooking spray

- 1 tbsp olive oil

- 2 6" corn tortillas

- 1 ½ cup cooked chicken breast

- 1 tomato

- 8 garlic cloves

- 2 chili peppers, Serrano is best

- ½ cup onion

Directions:

1. Preheat the oven to a temperature of 400°F.

2. Finely cut the cilantro and onion and mince the cloves of garlic.

3. Thinly dice the chilies and chop the tomato in two. Drop the skin and seeds and shred the bird.

4. Place the tortillas on a baking tray and break them into thin pieces. Using oil to spray and bake for about 3 min. Leave on to one side to cool.

5. Steam the oil until the onion has become transparent and sauté the onion, chilies and garlic.

6. Add the chicken, tomato, broth, and salt and then drop the bay leaf into the mixture.

7. Simmer for around 8 to 10 min and then incorporate the lime juice and cilantro. Season with pepper, taste and, if necessary, incorporate more lime.

8. With the tortilla sprinkled over the end, serve sweet.

37. Carrot and Coriander Soup

Serves: 4

Prep time: 3-5 min

Cooking time: 15 min

Ingredients:

- Freshly ground black pepper.

- Large bunch fresh coriander or fresh parsley, roughly chopped.

- (optional)

- 1 bay leaf

- 1.2 1/2 pints vegetable stock such as low salt Bouillon

- 1 tsp ground coriander

- 450g (1lb) carrots, sliced

- 1 onion, sliced

- 1 tbsp of vegetable or olive oil

Directions:

1. In a wide skillet, heat the oil and add the onions and carrots. Cook for 3-4 min before softening starts.

2. Stir in the cilantro from the field and season well. 1 min to cook.

3. Add in the bay leaf and vegetable stock and put it to a simmer. Simmer until soft with the vegetables.

4. Drop the bay leaf and use a hand processor or a blender to whizz the soup until creamy.

5. In a clean skillet, reheat, stir in the fresh cilantro or parsley and serve with some crusty bread.

38. Old Fashioned Pancakes

Serves: 2

Prep time: 3 min

Cooking time: 5-10 min

Ingredients:

- 1 tbsp vegetable oil

- ¼ cup of water

- ¼ cup 2% milk plus

- ¼ tsp baking powder

- ¼ cup granulated sugar

- 1 egg, beaten

- ½ cup all-purpose flour

Directions: In a pot, combine the first four ingredients. Mix thoroughly. Add water and milk. For thinner pancakes, add more water or, for thicker pancakes, fewer.Heat some oil in a pan or on a griddle. Pour on the griddle with ¼ cup of batter. Cook until brown, with each side twisted.

39. Cinnamon Tortilla Chips

Serves: 6

Prep time: 15 min

Cooking time: 10 min

Ingredients:

- 3 (6-inch) flour tortillas

- Pinch ground nutmeg

- ½ tsp ground cinnamon

- 2 tsp granulated sugar

- Cooking spray, for coating the tortillas

Directions:

1. Preheat your oven to about 350°F.

2. Line the parchment paper with a baking sheet.

3. Stir together the butter, cinnamon, and nutmeg in a small cup.

4. Lay the tortillas on a clean work surface and gently brush with cooking spray on both sides of each one.

5. Sprinkle each tortilla with the cinnamon sugar equally on both sides.

6. Break each of the tortillas into 16 wedges and placed them on the baking sheet.

7. Bake the tortilla wedges, rotating once, for around 10 min or until they are crisp.

8. Cool the chips and place them for up to 1 week at room temperature in a sealed bag.

40. Tuna Salad Bagel

Serves: 1

Prep time: 10 min

Cooking time: None

Ingredients:

- 1 bagel

- 1 lettuce leaf

- 1 tbsp mayonnaise, low-calorie

- 1 tbsp celery

- 1 tbsp onion

- ½ cup canned tuna with water, low-sodium

Directions:

1. Split the tuna into tiny bits.Finely chop the celery and onion. Combine the mayonnaise with the onion, celery, and tuna and combine properly. Put one part of the bagel with the lettuce leaf and scatter the mixture over before finishing off with the other half.

41. Chicken Soup

Serves: 4

Prep time: 10 min

Cooking time: 10 min

Ingredients:

- A squeeze of lemon juice

- 3 tbsp Greek yogurt or double cream

- 1 leek

- 300g (10½oz) leftover roast chicken, shredded and skin removed

- 1 tbsp cornflower (if required, see below)

- 1-liter low salt chicken stock

- 2 medium potatoes, peeled

- 3 medium carrots

- 1 tbsp of vegetable or olive oil

Directions:

1. Chop the carrots, leeks, and potatoes finely and cook until soft in a big pot of water.

2. Drain (do not recycle the cooking water) the vegetables and potatoes, transfer to the pot and add the stock.

3. Using a mixer to mix the soup to the consistency you want.

4. If you want to make the soup thicker: place the pan on low heat in the hob, combine the cornflower with a touch of cold water and add it to the soup.

5. Stir constantly until the broth thickens when simmering. Add in the chicken and leave for 5 min to cook.

6. Add the yogurt or cream and the lemon juice to the end.

42. French toast

Serves: 1

Prep time: 5 min

Cooking time: 5 min

Ingredients:

- 1 tbsp margarine

- ¼ tsp allspice

- ½ tsp cinnamon

- ¼ cup 1% milk

- 4 slices white bread (maybe toasted)

- 4 large egg whites, slightly beaten

Directions:

1. For egg whites, add in the cinnamon, milk, and allspice.

2. One slice at a time, dip the bread into the batter. Place it on a hot grill or in a molten margarine pan. Switch the bread around after it's golden brown. Serve hot with fructose (if diabetic, sugar-free.)

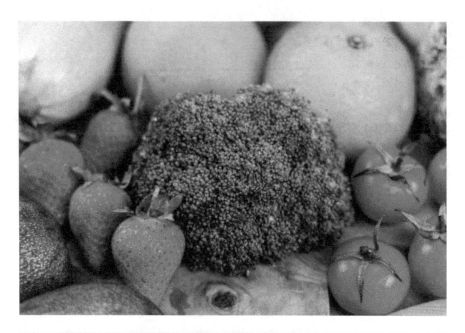

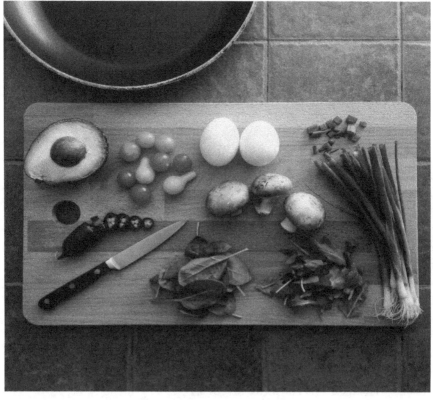

Chapter 4: Desserts

43. Rice Pudding

Serves: 6

Prep time: 15 min

Cooking time: 20 min

Ingredients:

- ½ tsp vanilla extract, or to taste

- 4 tbsp sugar

- 800ml soya milk (we used unsweetened)

- ¼ tsp nutmeg powder (optional)

- ½ tsp salt

- 200g (7oz) pudding rice

- ¼ tsp cinnamon powder (optional)

Directions:

1. In a wide skillet, add the soy milk and rice and mix as you get it to a boil.

2. Reduce the heat after boiling and cook for 20 min or until the rice is very tender.

3. Connect the butter, vanilla extract and salt, and roast stirring regularly for another 2 min.

4. Pour the rice pudding into serving plates and, if used, dust with nutmeg or cinnamon.

5. Serve instantly (hot) or cool down the rice pudding and serve it cold.

44. Tropical Vanilla Snow Cone

Serves: 4

Prep time: 15 min plus freezing time

Cooking time: None

Ingredients:

- 1 tbsp vanilla extract

- 2 tbsp granulated sugar

- 6 tbsp water

- 1 cup of frozen strawberries

- 1 cup pineapple

- 1 cup canned peaches

Directions:

1. Stir together the pineapple, peaches, strawberries, water and sugar in a wide saucepan over medium-high heat and bring to a simmer.

2. Lower the heat and let the mixture boil, stirring regularly, for 15 min.

3. Remove from the heat and allow to fully cooling the mixture for around 1 hour.

4. Move the fruit mixture to a food processor or blender and whisk in the vanilla.

5. Purée until smooth, then dump a 9x13 inch glass baking dish into the purée.

6. Cover and put the dish overnight in the fridge.

7. Using a fork to remove the sorbet until you have flaked colored ice while the fruit mixture is fully frozen.

8. Scoop the flakes of ice into four dishes for serving.

45. Lemon-Lime Sherbet

Serves: 8

Prep time: 5 min plus 3 hours chilling time

Cooking time: 15 min

Ingredients:

- ½ cup heavy (whipping) cream

- Juice of 1 lime

- Zest of 1 lime

- ½ cup freshly squeezed lemon juice

- 3 tbsp lemon zest, divided

- 1 cup granulated sugar

- 2 cup of water

Directions:

1. Over medium-high heat, put a wide saucepan and add the water, sugar, and two tbsp of the lemon's zest.

2. Bring the mixture to a boil and then reduce the fire for 15 min and simmer.

3. Place the mixture in a big bowl and add one tbsp of lemon zest, lemon juice, lime zest, and lime juice to the remaining mixture.

4. Chill the mixture in the fridge for around 3 hours before it is absolutely cold.

5. Whisk and pass the mixture to an ice cream machine with the heavy cream.

6. Freeze according to Directions: from the supplier.

46. Cherry Cake

Serves: 24

Prep time: 10-20 min

Cooking time: 45 min

Ingredients:

- 20 oz pie filling – cherry

- 1 tsp baking soda

- 1 tsp baking powder

- 1 tsp vanilla

- 2 cup white flour

- 1 cup sour cream

- 1 cup of sugar

- 2 eggs

- ½ cup butter, unsalted

Directions:

1. Preheat the oven to about 350°F and, at room temperature, soften the butter.

2. Cream together the eggs, sugar, vanilla, and sour cream.

3. Combine the baking powder, flour, and baking soda together in another dish.

4. Mix the dry ingredients progressively into the wet creamed mixture, folding to fully blend. Grease a 9x13 inch pan and dump the batter into it.

5. Layer the cherry mixture equally over the batter.

6. Bake for approximately 40 min, until golden brown.

47. Syrup Sponge Pudding

Serves: 4

Prep time: 15-20 min

Cooking time: 35-40 min

Ingredients:

- 6 tbsp golden syrup

- 100g (3½oz) self-rising flour

- 2 eggs

- 100g (3½oz) caster sugar

- 100g (3½oz) softened unsalted butter

Directions:

1. In a pot or food processor, cream the butter and sugar together.

2. To avoid curdling, add one egg and combine it gently with a spoon of flour. Add in the other egg and combine thoroughly.

3. Fold the flour in.

4. Measure the sugar into a bowl of buttered pudding. On top of the sugar, spoon the cake mixture on top.

5. With a fold, cover with buttered foil to allow for expansion.

6. Bake for 35-40 min at 200°C/400°F until a skewer comes out clean.

48. Tart Apple Granita

Serves: 4

Prep time: 15 min plus 4 hours freezing time

Cooking time: None

Ingredients:

- ¼ cup freshly squeezed lemon juice

- 2 cup unsweetened apple juice

- ½ cup of water

- ½ cup granulated sugar

Directions:

1. Warm the sugar and water in a medium-size saucepan over a medium-high flame.

2. Bring the mix to a boil and then decrease the flame to low and simmer for approximately 15 min more or until the liquid has halved.

3. Remove the pan from the flame and pipe the liquid into a big shallow metal pan.

4. For around 30 min, let the mixture settle and then mix in the apple juice and lemon juice.

5. In a freezer, put your pan.

6. Run a fork thru the fluid after 1 hour to break away any ice crystals that have developed. Scrape the sides off as well.

7. Put the pan back in the freezer and continue the stirring and scraping, making slush every 20 min.

8. Serve once; the mix is fully frozen and appears like crushed ice after around 3 hours.

49. Honey Bread Pudding

Serves: 4

Prep time: 15-20 min

Cooking time: 40-45 min

Ingredients:

- 6 cup cubed white bread

- 1 tsp pure vanilla extract

- ¼ cup honey

- 2 large egg whites

- 2 eggs

- 1½ cup plain rice milk

Directions:

1. Lightly oil a buttery, 8x8 inch baking dish; set aside.

2. Whisk the rice milk, eggs, egg whites, sugar, and vanilla together in a medium dish.

3. Add in the cubes of bread and mix until they are covered with the bread.

4. Move the mixture and cover with plastic wrap to the baking dish.

5. Hold the dish in the fridge for a minimum of 3 hours.

6. Preheat the oven to 325°F.

7. Remove the plastic wrap from the baking dish and bake the pudding for 35 to 40 min, or until the knife inserted in the middle comes out clean and golden brown.

8. Serve it hot.

50. Vanilla-Infused Couscous Pudding

Serves: 4

Prep time: 15-20 min

Cooking time: 20 min

Ingredients:

- 1 cup couscous

- ¼ tsp ground cinnamon

- ½ cup honey

- 1 vanilla bean, split

- ½ cup of water

- 1½ cup plain rice milk

Directions:

1. In a wide saucepan, combine the water, rice milk, and vanilla beans over medium to low heat.

2. Carry the milk to a gentle boil, reduce the flame to low, and let the milk simmer for around 10 min to enable the vanilla flavor to incorporate into the milk.

3. Remove the casserole from the flame.

4. Take the vanilla bean out and remove the seeds from the pod into the warm milk with the tip of a sharp knife.

5. Stir in the cinnamon and sugar.

6. Cover the plate, stir in the couscous, and let sit for about 10 min.

7. With a fork, before eating, fluff the couscous.

51. Victoria Sponge Cake

Serves: 4

Prep time: 10 min

Cooking time: 35 min

Ingredients:

- 50ml double cream

- A splash of milk (if required)

- 250g (9oz) self-rising flour

- 4 medium eggs

- 250g (9oz) caster sugar

- 250g (9oz) unsalted butter, well softened

- Approximately 5 tbsp raspberry jam (add more or less for your preferred taste)

Directions:

1. Grease two 20cm shallow cake tins, and then line them with parchment for baking. Preheat the oven to 180°C/350°F.

2. In a wide cup, incorporate the melted butter and sugar and beat until really pale and fluffy. It is likely that this would take about 5-10 min. This can be achieved in a free-standing mixer if needed.

3. Add to the mixture an egg and a giant spoon of flour and beat again. Until all the eggs are incorporated, repeat this process. Sift the excess flour in, and then use a broad metal spoon to fold onto the mixture.

4. Add a splash of milk if the paste does not have a falling consistency (i.e., it quickly slips off a spoon).

5. Break the mixture between the two tins, smooth the surface, and bake 25 min in the oven.

6. They should be sandwiched together until the cakes have been boiled and cooled. Whisk the double cream until soft peaks form. Spread the jelly on top of one of the cakes and then spread the whipped cream on top of the jam. Sit on top of the second cake and sift through the icing sugar for decoration.

Conclusion

We want to encourage you to take the time to read this book because we hope it has enabled you to learn what the kidney diet is all about and because if you have been diagnosed with kidney failure, you should adopt it.

Before you follow the renal diet, we advise you to obtain medical guidance, and your healthcare professional may need to inform you how much potassium, sodium, etc. you are going to be eating. And, of course, you'll need to adopt a specific diet entirely while you're on the dial.

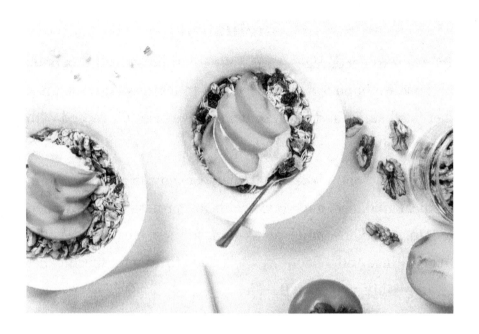

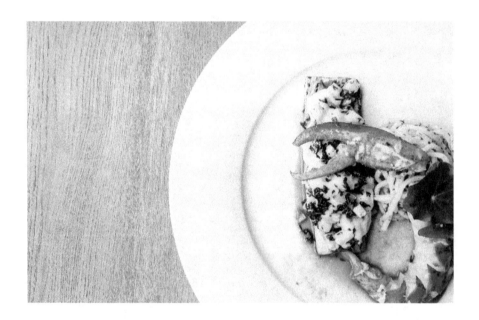